EPILEPSY
and
All the Torments

by
Joanne Curry

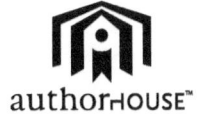

authorHOUSE™

1663 LIBERTY DRIVE, SUITE 200
BLOOMINGTON, INDIANA 47403
(800) 839-8640
WWW.AUTHORHOUSE.COM

AuthorHouse™
1663 Liberty Drive, Suite 200
Bloomington, IN 47403
www.authorhouse.com
Phone: 1-800-839-8640

AuthorHouse™ UK Ltd.
500 Avebury Boulevard
Central Milton Keynes, MK9 2BE
www.authorhouse.co.uk
Phone: 08001974150

This book is a work of non-fiction. Unless otherwise noted, the author
and the publisher make no explicit guarantees as to the accuracy
of the information contained in this book and in some cases, names
of people and places have been altered to protect their privacy.

First published by AuthorHouse 2/13/2006

ISBN: 1-4208-8785-8 (sc)

Printed in the United States of America
Bloomington, Indiana

This book is printed on acid-free paper.

Contents

Introduction

Epilepsy: It is not just about having seizures and when the seizures are over with, and all of a suddenly everything is okay. Comedians are continuously cracking jokes about epileptics and seizures.

On two certain occasions, I was watching a certain game show and a movie (no names mentioned). On the game show a certain category was titled "Are you dancing or having a seizure"? The audience and contestants all burst out laughing. In regards to the movie, these two men were talking and one of the men was describing a certain female. He was "scrunching his body" while describing her saying she was "so fine". The other male (a friend) whom was listening asked if she was "epileptic". It was obvious the one that said "the epileptic" was trying to be funny. In fact he mentioned "the epileptic" twice. The listening friend knew exactly what his friend was talking about when he was scrunching his body around (she was one sexy lady!).

I had status epilepsy (the worse kind as they occur more often). It is more than anything, a lack of misunderstanding of the medical illness and all its torments that come along with the package.

I want to be able to help epileptics (in anyway I can) and get a lot of doctors and others to realize how serious epilepsy is. Please understand I'm not just mocking all doctors or people, I only mean about what I went through. After 46 years of experiencing seizures, I pretty much know of what I'm writing about. With short-term memory loss and brain damage from the multitude of seizures I had, I did the best I could (I'll reveal more personal stuff later on).

I am sure a lot of things will probably change in my life after all of this is written. I may even start having many seizures again. If that happens, I just pray that they do not occur as often or as violent as those I have had in my past, before I had brain surgery. It would be a dream come true for me to appear on the Montel Williams Show and maybe even go so far as to have a movie made of my life and all that I have gone through (I wonder what two professional actresses would want to play my role? That as when I was a child. That as an adult?).

My goal is not to see if I can write the great all-American novel or even a large book. My goal is to get my messages across to the whole world (I want to be proof that other epileptics might need to get other people to understand some of what an epileptic goes through in this life).

God Bless You All Richly.

x

Chapter 1
My Early Childhood

This chapter will not be very long due to my lack of memory caused by the numerous seizures I've had in my life. According to my mother I had my first seizure when I was only two (2) years of age. I had gone into a coma for one week and my body was hard as dried cement due to that seizure.

The first neurosurgeon who ever examined me told my mother I had a bruise on the left side of my brain. I had kept on having seizures, but back in the 1950's, they didn't have knowledge about seizures then as they have now. It had also been said to my mother by my family physician that I was "allergic to eggs". The allergic to the eggs business sounds like a medical guess to me. I've eaten eggs throughout my life and do not feel that I am allergic to them. The business of the bruise in the brain and being allergic to eggs is a big difference in medical diagnosis. After one week of being comatose my body started to "defrost". Even though I finally came out of the coma, I was still having seizures. I had the grand mal type, as most epileptic knows, we get "aura feelings". With me personally, I rather have the actual convulsion than the aura feeling. The convulsions would hit me as fast as lightning strikes. With the aura feelings, mine were very slow and dragged out. Who would want something so horrible to last so long?

This sounds cold, but it is the easiest way to explain it. This is how the aura feelings felt (at least with me). Imagine a police officer comes up to you and tells you your beloved child has just been murdered. Can you imagine how you would feel as a parent? I am a mother, I would know how awful that would feel. Well, the 'aura.feeling' (again, I am describing myself, not everyone) is about 1,100 times more intensified (or they are for me when I have a seizure).

I honestly do not know how else to describe it. One thing I know for sure without a doubt, I am not exaggerating. Most of us epileptics are tormented more than anyone can ever understand. I pray with all my heart that once this book is completed with our Lord Jesus' help, that there will be a lot better understanding. Jesus, I ask you to richly bless everyone who helps me with my book, all the readers too. Guide them with your amazing knowledge and with the Holy Spirit guiding them.

Speaking of childhood, I have a friend who has a child approximately 19 years of age. This friend told me one time that her child had twelve seizures daily for seventeen straight years. As crazy as some people might find this to believe, I have no doubt that what she told me is true. What I mean is why not at times just eleven seizures or thirteen, but why they were always twelve on a daily basis? That is how weird and unpredictable seizures can be. I thank God with all my heart that this friends' child finally stopped having seizures. It does not matter how they stopped, just that they did stop. So as crazy as things sound concerning epilepsy, do not be surprised about all you read or hear from others or myself with anything having to do with seizures.

 In your loving name Jesus.

(Thank-you Lord)

Chapter 2
The Agony of Being in School

One of the things that triggered by brain into going into seizures would be fear. Being that it was the first time in school and being only five years old, naturally I had plenty of fear. I might as well say my school education never ever got accomplished. Every time I turned around I was having seizures.

Whether in kindergarten or a higher grade, how can you do school work when you're unconscious and not aware of what is going on around you? While still in elementary, I remember lots of times when I woke up from unconsciousness I would be getting spanked with the teacher's ruler. It's hard to believe, but true (even now epilepsy is very hard to understand, much less way back in the late 1950's and early 1960's).

So, I've gotten even older. Now I am in junior high school (middle school today). Oh my sweet Lord Jesus, I could have had never made it without you. In junior high school, it was pure hell for me. It seemed like I was forever awakening from being unconscious. Can you even began to imagine how embarrassing it was for me to wake up and find myself covered with urination from wetting myself while having the seizure? All my former classmates (and other students that were not my classmates) were continuously making fun of me. After school, I remembered getting off the bus and walking home, all seemed to be going well, and then the next thing I knew I would be waking up on the side of the road. The other students would be kicking me on each side of my ribs. Why always on each side of my ribs, I didn't know then and have never gotten an answer why they did so.

I remember I had only one true friend. Her name was Frances. I loved her dearly then as my friend and still do. I had so many seizures; the school office staff started getting "suspicious". It was in the 1960's, with drugs like heroin, LSD and the other illicit drugs that were so popular then. I remember one-time I was in the principals' office and my mother was called to come and get me because of me having had a seizure. The principals' office staff had a bad argument with my mother over me even being in school. Since drugs were popular then, as far as the school was concerned, illicit drugs were why I was 'acting' so weird, not because I was having a seizure or seizures. My mother would be screaming out to them "No, she's not on drugs!" It didn't matter what notes the doctor(s) wrote, what records he sent, or whatever my mother tried to convince the school staff, the staff still would not believe that was why I was having seizures because I was doing drugs and did not have epliepsy. The school administration thought that even if I had epilepsy, to them I could not possibly have that many seizures (again, this was what they felt, but not what the doctor tried to tell them).

Due to all of my convulsions, it affected my memory something terrible. I was in the middle of ninth grade and I couldn't stand it any longer so I just quit school. What was I accomplishing? With my memory being poor (because of having so many seizures) I always made bad grades. I would learn something and know it real well to begin with, but my mind would go blank when I tried recalling them. I had always enjoyed school itself and I truly loved to learn things. I was always one who had to ask questions. (I still do even now). Leave it up to my seizures to start to ruin my life.

I absolutely had no plans to quit school, it just turned out that way. Later on in years (after marriage to my second husband I have now) I started taking GED classes. I not only wanted to learn, but it would also give me something to do. So, I enrolled and started in adult GED classes. It was a joyful time to me, I loved it being in class and being able to learn once again. After I had started classes, which were being held downstairs in the building that the class was held, the facility started having other students coming in and they were physically handicapped (walkers, canes, wheelchairs, etc.). Because of them being handicapped, they took over our class downstairs and my former classroom was moved upstairs. (Oh, I had immediately told my teacher when school first started that I had seizures). Even though I could walk with no problems, this teacher told me I had to stay downstairs in another classroom by myself, not with the other special needy students (you probably guessed why). The teacher could not take the chance of me having a seizure either going up or down the stairs. I came out and asked her: "How am I suppose to learn in another classroom all by myself? What about when I have questions, what am I suppose to do, scream out and ask her questions from downstairs? How am I supposed to copy notes off the chalkboard?" No matter how hard I tried to get this teacher to allow me to go upstairs, I couldn't get her to change her mind. I never could figure out why she just didn't have the whole class move into the other classroom downstairs. Believe me, I kept asking her why we couldn't take the other classroom downstairs, but she never would tell me why. So, here we go again, I had to quit. What other choice did I have? I felt totally abandoned and isolated.

Plenty of time went by and after my brain surgery I thought I would try again with the GED classes. I walked down to the school and it was closed (not just for the day, but closed as far as no classes were open). I started praying to our Lord Jesus about it. It was only about one week later I went by there again and read the sign on the side of the building for the GED classes. I was so happy, Jesus answered another prayer! Well, I went to get registered and then I found out that the GED class was only at night because the day time classes was only for students who wanted to learn english. Well, I already know english.

I also did not want to go to the GED classes at night, I wanted to be in church instead (my present church now not only has their door opened for services on Sunday's, but also on Monday, Tuesday, Wednesday, Thursday and Friday evenings). Well, it was time to talk to Jesus again. I kept asking Jesus over and over: "Why Lord, why? Lord" I had been praying for the classes to start again. They did, and I thought for sure that I would be able to get back in school and work on my GED. I was so disappointed I started to get depressed. I immediately thought of the bible scriptures: "My ways, My thoughts are not your ways, your thoughts" (Isaiah, 55, verses 8-9). Then all of a sudden the Lord spoke to me that I deeply desired to write a book about my life. I had no time for school. I had to get started on this book.

Writing this book, helping others in anyway I can, means more to me than a GED class. I thank God now, I understand now. God had a better plan ahead for me! Thank you sweet loving Jesus. I praise you, and give you glory and honor. I have had to learn to trust in Jesus no matter how bad things looked. I could not make it without prayers and Jesus. I am truly guided by his Holy Spirit.

Chapter 3
Worktime

I remember the first job I ever had. I was 13 years old. I went to work at a childcare center after school. The childcare center was right across the street from where I lived, so I would just walk there.

Since the owners knew I had seizures, I was absolutely not allowed to pick up the babies in the day care center (which was certainly understandable). I mainly worked with the older children. Now, if a baby was already in their crib, I could do things like, change their diapers or clothes, hand them a bottle (the older babies could handle the bottles on their own), as obviously there was no reason to pick them up.

Another job I had was working in a place that sold mobile homes. I would do things like going in all of the mobile homes and dust, pick up any trash that people would leave behind, etc. After all everything would have to be clean and look it best for a sale. I know that was my favorite job because it was unique to me. Why? Inside all the mobile homes had price tags on each of the items that were in the home (mainly items like pictures on the walls, floral arrangements on the tables, etc...). If a customer was in one of the mobile homes, but didn't want to buy it, yet wanted to purchase a picture on the wall, they could purchase it for whatever the price tag indicated. If a picture was sold, it was part of my job to get another like it from the warehouse and put it where the other picture was. If the warehouse did not have the same picture, then it was up to me to choose whichever one I wanted to get. I really loved that part of it, because I learned to decorate and it taught me to decorate my own living environment when I got to living on my own and when I got married, as I continue to do now.

This job was so far away from where I lived that I had to quit because of my not being able to drive and having to get someone to give me a ride. The individual got tired of taking me. I never told them in the beginning that I had seizures. I thank God nothing ever happened. I had to have someway to get some money to survive. There were bills I had to pay like everyone else.

When I was around 30 years old, I got a job at a retirement home. I really also enjoyed that job. It made me feel so good inside to help the elderly, handicapped children and animals. My former boss, knew of my seizures, but she allowed me to work there because my mother also worked there with me.

There were other jobs in between that I applied for, and at times, I would tell them I had seizures. Lots of jobs wouldn't even allow me to do volunteer work there, much less get paid for it. Most of the employers were terrified that if they hired me and I went into a convulsion and got injured that I would file a lawsuit against them. I would never do that, but I clearly understood why they 'had' to do this. It did hurt whenever they would not hire me because of my seizures.

I would have had been happy enough just to be given a chance. At my husbands' job, once in awhile they would allow me to do volunteer work when they would need me. Since my surgery I have done minor things like help out my husband's secretary while she has a day off or was on vacation. I would go in and answer the telephone for her. I would just transfer a call through a workers phone line or if a particular worker was not in their office, I would simply take a message.

I can speak spanish. Many times people have used me to interpret for them. I have done this in a restaurant and have done so also while sitting in a hospital lobby. That's enjoyable, but my main goal now is getting this book completed. I don't think I can ever stop thanking Jesus of his plans for me. Lean not toward thy own understating, but Trust thy Lord with all thy heart (Proverbs, 3, verse 5).

Speaking of work, I highly recommend that everyone, especially epileptics watch the movie "Bone Collector" with Denzel Washington. Even though it is not a true story, Denzel does an excellent role of acting as a bed-bound police detective who becomes a quadriplegic who has seizures. He is still able to come to grips with his health issues and able to solve crimes. In watching this movie it helped me realize (though I know it was just a movie) that even with all of his problems he was able to overcome his handicap and still use his mind to solve crime. There are many people with handicaps that do work and on a daily basis their work contributes to the betterment of mankind. I see people whom some people would not believe capable of working work and do quality jobs. I admire them and so should all of us.

Chapter 4
Medical Theories/injuries

When I became an adult it was a real trial to deal with medical personnel (this was before I met my current neurologist and neurosurgeon). In 1982 I lived in South Carolina. The doctor I was seeing there had me on Dilantin. I was taking it in 100 milligram dosages at 3 capsules per day. This former doctor took a Dilantin blood level test on me. He told me: "With as much Dilantin as you are on, your Dilantin level should read a point 12, your level only reads a point 2". Immediately, he accused me of not taking my medicine as he had prescribed. I came out and told him that I could not afford to pay for doctor appointments, office visits, special tests, medications, hospital bills, etc., and not to adhere to any medication that a doctor prescribed. Him telling me this enraged me.

Then when an EEG test was taken, it always came out "normal". I would ask them, "How did you expect it to come out? I did not have a seizure during the test. They would all look at me like I was crazy. Even when I was pregnant with my daughter Jennifer Marie, I was taking 1,050 milligrams of Dilantin and mysoline daily and the level checks came out low. I told them that I did not like taking that much while I was pregnant, but I did not like having the seizures, either. I could not win whether I was on a small or large amount of medication.

One time I went to the emergency room because of my having a multitude of seizures one after another. When I arrived there, I already told them I took my medicine before I had left home. They took a Phenobarbital (which was the medication I was on at that time) blood level test and it came out low (I already warned them because of my experience with Dilantin). The nurse gave me two more Phenobarbital pills and took another blood level test. How do you think it came out? Yes, you probably guess right- it came out low. Then I was given more Phenobarbital through the IV directly into my blood stream. They checked me again and guess what, this check was also indicated a low level of the medication.

The emergency room immediately called my family physician. He had ordered a liver test and the liver test came out "okay". The emergency room nurse told me her own daughter had been going through the same thing as I was. Whatever reason her daughter was on a medication for, it would not also show up in her blood. Then her daughter was also being accused of not taking her medication. Her mother, the nurse, said, "Oh yes, she is taking her medicine, I watch her take it to make sure!"

I had kept telling myself something is wrong. When I meet my current neurosurgeon, I told him what the family physician had said about me taking my medication as he had prescribed and the neurosurgeon said: "Oh no, sometimes if your liver works too fast (like rejecting my medicine) it can be considered a bad liver". It turned out that my metabolism works really fast. I was once on an anticonvulsant and was having a lot of seizures and my dentures were rotting, my hair was falling out in great big blobs and the doctor told me I was having an allergic reaction to the medication for seizures that he had prescribed for me. I ended up going to the emergency room because of so many seizures while on the anticonvulsant.

One doctor I was seeing asked me what were the medications I had already tried. I was naming one medication after another real fast. When I mentioned one medication that I had taken in the past, he immediately spoke to me in a sarcastic manner and told me: "Oh, that medication has not even come out on the market yet". I said: "Oh really, why don't you contact the doctor that wrote out the prescription?. Why don't you also call the drug store that filled the prescription?" The doctor just turned around and walked out. The doctor knew he could not out-smart me. There was absolutely no reason for him to act so hateful towards me.

One time I had a seizure and I got severely burned. As far as the hospital was concerned I was faking it to get attention. This is what happened: I had a four quart pot and which was fairly full of water which I was heating to make some iced tea to have for later. After the water came to a full boil the last thing I remember was turning off the stove. I had a seizure right after that apparently. When I was convulsing, my hand must of had been jerking up and down and caused it to hit the side of the pot, with caused it to turn over onto me. I woke up on the kitchen floor and there was water everywhere. I called my family doctor, and his nurse told me to splatter cold water all over me and call the paramedics. The paramedic's arrived and when we got to the hospital, one of them called my husband at work to tell him of what happened. He told my husband specifically that I had to have been unconscious before I even fell to the floor, because no human being could take that kind of pain (from the boiling water).

Whether I was unconscious before I fell to the floor, or after, I do not recall. All I know for sure I was able to take the pain because Jesus was with me. When the paramedics arrived they found me waiting quietly outside the front door to our home. They expected to find me screaming my head off in pain.

I was kind of woozy from just waking up from being unconsciousness, which upon reflection probably helped me not to feel much of the pain at that point in time.

I remember one the paramedics trying to take off my blouse without even pouring saline on me. Oh my, I really did scream my head off then. I kept screaming out: "pour saline on me, pour saline on me". The blouse was stuck to my skin and his trying to remove it from me was causing me to be in a lot of pain as he was also taking layers of my skin off along with the blouse (the skin had adhered to the blouse). If he had used the saline to begin with, all that pain could have had easily been avoided and my blouse removed without so much difficulty. The paramedic ended up using six pints just to loosen up my blouse and remove it from my body. I had first, second and third degree burns across my chest area.

Do you know what it is like to have your body turn so hard from a seizure that an IV cannot be even inserted into your body (my gosh)? When I have a seizure my body has become so rigid that medical personnel have not even been able to insert an IV into me.

Another time I fell into a ditch (from a seizure) and I received a smashed knee, broken leg and a compound fractured ankle (all on my left side). I ended up with a plate and seven pins and of coarse had to have a cast put on. In fact, one of the pins came unscrewed and was trying to pop out through my ankle (it felt like a sharp knife trying to pierce through). I figured the tip part of it was trying to get through. I told the doctor who had operated on me what was happening and he refused to believe me. He said that the pins do not come unscrewed. Bull! Apparently it turned around because it eventually did come out head-first just like a baby. When I had called the doctor's office to tell him, I was told to go into his office immediately. As the male nurse was using the tweezers to take out the pin out of my ankle, he was trying to be funny. He was telling me 'Oh Joanne, I knew you had a loose screw somewhere". I personally did not think it was funny. I knew what he was trying to do (not say the doctor was wrong about the pin not coming out of my ankle) so that I would not sue the doctor (which I did not).

In having seizure, many times I have stopped breathing to where I turned blue from lack of oxygen. One other time I had a seizure and went falling straight back landing on my tailbone. I ended up with a fractured tailbone. After this I would have to lean all the way to the left or right side when sitting down, and would have to mainly sit on my hips which was extremely painful to me. Another time I had another seizure and landed flat on my back which caused me to have a pinched nerve and get a disc in my back out of place.

Out of all my different (and may I add, I am only speaking of the ones that I remember) injuries, the back injury was the most painful. I had no pain in my back then, also, because an extreme amount of pain went down my left leg. Several months went by and I still had a bruise on my back. I could not help to be curious about that, so I asked the doctors I was seeing: "why?" (an orthopedic and chiropractic). The chiropractic said I should not lose sleep over it. Then he went on to tell me that I was probably still bleeding inside. I thought "Bleeding?" The chiropractic doctor had to pop the nerve/disc back into place. I remember before then, that I had begged and begged the orthopedic doctor to cut off my leg. I was very serious. I could hardly stand the pain. He never would though and now I am so thankful.

On another occasion I was walking on the sidewalk going to my girlfriends' place of business. The next thing I knew I was waking up lying on my back. All I saw was 'blurry' people and they looked like men. I got scarred and immediately started to ask them over and over who they were. They told me they were the paramedics. I was still scared, so I kept asking for my husband because of me being so afraid. One paramedic told me he was already there. I guess I passed out again because when I woke up the next time, I was in the hospital. After the emergency staff had examined me they found out I had a cut on the back of my head because of me falling. My falling onto the asphalt on the side of the road had caused a cut to open. Wow, on the hard pavement you could just imagine how painful that was! After that I had awakened to find the nurse cleaning out all of the blood from my hair and scalp. It took a long time for her to finally get me all cleaned up. She was then able to see the wound better.

The nurse came out and told me: "You cannot stop bleeding" which for some reason immediately made me throw up (it looked like to me like nothing but water). It reminded me of a balloon that is filled with water, tied in a knot and thrown on the ground real hard. You know how forceful it comes out? That is how forceful that water came flying out of my mouth. The nurse went out to get the doctor, but came back in alone.

The nurse told me that I was going home. I was not ashamed or embarrassed by what I did next. I immediately started quoting out loud the Holy Bible scripture Ezekiel 16:6 (When I passed by thee, I saw thee polluted in thy own blood, I said unto thee why waste thy blood, live,₁ I say live). Right then and there my bleeding stopped.

I have had to use that scripture other times in my personal life. I remember that scripture I learned way back in 1976. I pray to God that I will never forget it. I remember the first time I learned Ezekiel 16:6. I was still living in South Carolina. I had a real good friend name Gwen. She was with these two brothers. One was about 5 and the other 7. They got into a fight and the younger boy bit the older boy. In fact, he bit him so hard that he actually put a hole in his brothers' arm! Gwen immediately started quoting the Ezekiel 16:6 scripture. As she was using the scripture, I remember I saw a real small white dot like inside his arm by his bone. No, the hole was not big enough to where I saw through the hole naturally. It was like a vision; all of a sudden the child's arm was completed covered with a new layer of skin!

That was the first miracle that I had ever seen. I was learning a lot of the Holy Spirit then too. It is amazing of what can happen. All you have to do is believe in Jesus! I remember then I praised God and gave him all the glory and honor and I still do.

Believe me, something like that you do not forget. Even if you doubt, what do you have to lose except a lot of blood. Why not try it? When I had to use it for myself, all I had to do is keep believing and Jesus blessed my faith. I had a former neurologist tell me that I was "Not having seizures, but anxiety attacks".

Good grief, I did not even finish high school and I had more common sense than that. With anxiety attacks you generally do not chew all the inside of your mouth, foam, have your body turn hard as dried cement, turn blue, go into a coma, etc.

It is really sad of how a lot of people (and even some doctors) do not even know about epilepsy. I had met a neurologist (out of town) in a hospital. They were able to see for themselves that my seizures would not stop. They called in the neurologist and he told me "Even though I am a neurologist, I am not qualified to take care of you. There is neurologist in Tampa I want you to see". I went to see that neurologist in Tampa, Florida and he ran seven tests on me and then recommended I have 'brain' surgery.

Usually when you need real special medical care, you end up in the bigger cities. How many of you epileptics have experienced all that I have been through? I kept telling our Lord Jesus that was one of the reasons I wanted to write this book. I want you to know it is not just you. You are not some freak and you are not alone. I clearly understand what all of you are going through. I know what the emotional and physical pain feels like; the rejections; the misunderstandings. I know what it feels like not to even be given a chance.

It is a blessing to have someone to relate to your problems. Besides writing this book, the most I can do is pray and pray to Jesus. He understands you more than anyone! I will go to meetings, talk shows, whatever it takes to make the world more knowledgeable. I am sure my neurosurgeon will get me involved in things. Oh concerning me "faking it to get attention", I could not fake it if I tried. I am not that low down. In fact, even if I tried to fake seizures, I would probably crack up laughing. It is not because it is funny, it is because I know I am not a professional actress. It is just not in me to fake a seizure.

Joanne Curry

Everyone that does not understand, need to know that it is a very serious and dangerous medical illness. Each seizure could possible kill someone. I would love to go back to my old school, doctor's offices and hospitals and let them know how wrong they were. Of course, they all have different workers by now, except for the same workers in some doctor's offices and hospitals. I bet a lot of them would be shocked to find out I had to end up with brain surgery.

It really would not be worth my time. Even though there is more understanding now, there still is not enough understanding. Will there ever be enough understanding? Probably not! Another time I was washing dishes and was alone in the house. As I was rinsing off a steak knife (the one with the sharp ridges across it) I went into a seizure. The next thing I knew, I was waking up in bed (I don't recall how I got there). I felt liquid going down the right side of my head. I thought: "It must be hot in here, I'm sweating." Then I got to thinking that it could not be hot, it's February. Then I realized what happened, recalling what I had been doing. I had to force myself to get out of bed to check myself. I finally managed to get into the bathroom and I looked in the mirror. I found a stab wound right in the middle of my forehead and right above my right eye. I found where I had been bleeding and somehow been using towels to soak up the blood (I have not been able to ever recall using the towels or how I got into bed). Can you imagine if I had accidentally stab myself in the eye? Again, I ended up going to the doctor who sent me to the hospital for seven stitches over my eye. Oh, eight stitches on my forehead.

I could not possibly remember all of my lifetime injuries, but I covered pretty much the major ones, that I am able to recall or someone has told me about. What was so sad and aggravating was most of the times I went into the emergency rooms, they would all look like: "What are we suppose to do with you?" All I can say is that I pray to Jesus that the medical knowledge will become even better.

With me, if I got pregnant, had a migraine headache, get overly tired, or even start to menstruate, anything seems to just about cause me to go into a seizure. Things that happen over and over again, are not all coincidences. These are the types of things that need to be learned about epileptics.

One time I felt the need to get into the shower for some strange reason. I had just taken one not long before I started feeling this way, so I was not dirty or did I need to take another one. For some reason I just kept feeling the need to get into the shower. I even asked Jesus over and over again because I did not know why I felt this great urge to get into the shower. After some soul searching and not finding an answer I went into the shower. I started taking a shower and was all wet and had soap all over my body and shampoo in my hair. Jesus spoke to me then and said: "Get out now, you are going to have a seizure." I did appreciate him telling me this, but I still wondered why he waited to tell me then and not earlier. I did ask the Lord to give me about ten seconds to rinse off the soap and shampoo. In our shower we have the showerhead that is attached to the hose with which you can use it as a regular shower head or use it with the hose. I quickly rinsed myself off and got out of the shower. I usually dry off with the towel in the bathroom, but for some reason on this occasion I had better go into the bedroom to dry off. I did not want to dry off in the bathroom and have the chance of having a seizure and go flying down into the bathtub and injuring myself or if there was still water in the tub, accidentally drowning. I ended off drying off in the bedroom, put my clothing on and went into the den. I turned on the television to distract what was going on in my mind and help the time go by quicker. Knowing I was going to have a seizure was extremely terrifying to me this time as it has been on numerous other occasions. All in all it took about twenty minutes for me to have the seizure. Waiting for something like that seemed to be twenty hours, especially being kept waiting and wanting for the feeling and attack to be over with. I recall screaming out: "Jesus, Jesus!" Next thing I recalled I was awakening from being unconscious.

I am sure a lot of people will think Satan was trying to get me into the shower so that I would drown. Yes, I admit he wants me dead as well as everyone else, but I believe the Lord Jesus was involved in this with all my heart. Why, do I believe it to be so? Because every since this incident with my feeling the need to take this particular shower and Jesus telling me to get out, now I can shower, cook, wash dishes, etc., alone without having anyone be in the home with me. I believe Jesus was trying to teach me not to have fear and to trust in him at all times. I live the best I can everyday since this time. I want everyone who has seizures out there to understand that I know what they are going through and what trial and tribulations they face. A lot of you may not have had it as serious as me and I know that there are other people who have it worse than I, but we do not need to be afraid any longer. Jesus is with each of us and will protect us from harm.

Remember, this is not all for medical personnel, it is for everyone who needs a better understanding of what anyone who might have seizures, no matter what the cause may be have to go through when they get sick.

In Your Holy name (Jesus, bless us all).

Jesus

Chapter 5
Where is the Christian Love?

As of right now, across the street from where I live there is a church. I use to go there because it was easy to just walk across the street. One particular day, I was visiting in the church and I went into a seizure. When I had awakened from being unconscious the pastor immediately started to tell me off. He came out and told me to get out of the church, that he did not want any "liability charges." He even went on to tell me: "And don't even come back to do volunteer work." (I had just offered to do volunteer work in the kitchen because they were planning for a get together a meal after the service).

I was hurt way deep down inside. I was still a little bit wobbly. A married couple helped me walk across the street back to my home. The more I recovered from the seizure, the more I thought about it over and over. I got so angry, I screamed out: "Jesus, if that is the so called Christian love, I do not want anything to do with it!" (Please, don't misunderstand me. I was not angry at Jesus, I was angry at the pastor). I fell into a very deep depression and ended up in a psychiatric unit. After I got back home again I thought of it more and more.

Just seeing the church right across the street would reminded me so easily all over again of what had happened. Then one particular day, I was just sitting in my lounge chair thinking over and over of what happened. I suddenly started screaming out over and over: "I hate all churches, I hate all pastors!" Oh how hurt and angry I was. All of a sudden our Lord Jesus spoke to me and said: "<u>You can't go around blaming all churches and all the pastors because of what happened</u>". I thought, "You're right Lord, you're right". I immediately picked up my telephone book and started looking for a new church to attend (Oh, before I go on, I was even told I was demon possessed). As I was going down the list, and as soon as I read Refuge Church of Our Lord (Pastor Ira J. McCloud) Jesus suddenly spoke to me and said: "Call that church". I did and I left a message. They returned my call in no time at all and they even came out to pick me up and took me to their church. (Note: God's voice is not spoken out loud. It is an inner voice. You must experience it to truly understand. It is a beautiful gift to hear).

At Refuge Church of Our Lord (Sebring, FL) with Pastor Ira J. McCloud is where I found true Christian love. Everyone is so kind and respectful. After I started attending Refuge Church of Our Lord (before I had my surgery) I started to have seizures again on a regular basis. They never kicked me out, especially my pastor. They all prayed for me to make sure Jesus took care of me. They have always acted concerned over me and shown great love and compassion to me. If I do not attend church for a while, they will either call or stop by to check up on me. They all have the true love of Jesus in them. If anyone calls on the phone, they always answer:

"Praise the Lord". They constantly give Jesus all the praise, glory and honor.

I could not make it myself without Jesus' help and without the help from the church. I have never even seen a church love the Lord as much as they do. Now I understand why the Lord spoke to me about calling the church. I can never thank the Lord enough for taking the time to speak to me about the church. Just about everything they do is religious related. They attend the church on Monday's, Wednesday's, Friday's and Sundays. Sometimes they will visit other churches on the rest of their week.

Refuge Church of Our Lord is an apostolic religion. They even wash each other's feet as Jesus said to do. It's in the book of John 13:14-15 "If I then, your Lord and Master, have washed your feet; ye also ought to wash one another's feet." They are always willing to help in anyway. When I had my surgery it was at a hospital two hours away from where I live. They were willing to drive a long distance to visit me. The church is mainly African-American, but that is fine. I have never been prejudice. As of right now, I am the only white woman there (I'm sure more will arrive in the future) and one white male (we are not married).

I really do enjoy myself with them, more than they can ever know. I look forward to attending church there. They help me build up my inner strength, along with the Lord's help. It is very obvious that God works through them as an instrument to help me. If I ever need to speak to anyone they are always ready to listen. If I need to cry, again they are there ready to listen.

They believe in divine healing, but they still go to the doctor. Whether they are healed divinely through Jesus or Jesus uses a doctor as an instrument, they always, I mean **_Always,_** give the Lord the praise, glory and honor.

Refuge Church of Our Lord also believes in unknown tongues. (I will write out bible scriptures later on). It is a small church, but you can certainly feel God's power and love in the church. Pastor Ira J. McCloud and his wife Mother Pirieta McCloud is considered our spiritual parents. The ministers and deacons are all called Minister or deacon (their first or last name). They prefer not to call each other by just their first names. This way more respect is shown (other churches I had already been to, they all called each other by their first name). Of course, whatever church, does their own way is their business. The ones without titles are simply called brother or sister (their first or last name).

At times after the church service, a few of us will go out to eat then return to church (some Sunday's it is from about 10:am — 10:00pm). There is fantastic preaching and great singing. Everyone is always smiling and happy. They leave everything in the Lord's hands.

It is utterly amazing of how strong they believe in Jesus. I'm so glad Lord Jesus that you spoke to me and said: "Call that church." I know there is some type of reason the Lord wants me there. Please speak to them Lord as they are reading this book (or even those who are not reading this) and tell them yourself of how much I love them, how much I appreciate them. I thank you

Lord Jesus; PRAISE BE TO THY MOST HOLY FATHER.

Concerning people with seizures being possessed by demons: For those of you reading this that believe that someone having a seizure please stop and think of this; If it is truly demons causing or doing this, then what about the persons who have their seizures under control, with the use of medications? Don't you think common sense would tell you that demons most likely have more 'power' than any medication available to mankind? If this were so, what good would medications be and how come they work for some individuals?

To visit the Church: Refuge Church of our Lord

> Pastor Ira J. McCloud
> 642 Harris Street
> Sebring, FL 33870-3071
> (863) 382-1855

Mailing Address: Refuge Church of our Lord

> P. O. Box 3831
> Sebring, FL 33870-3071

In your Name, Jesus

Chapter 6
Holy Bible Sciptures

• Job 28:28 - And unto man he said Behold, the fear of the Lord, that is wisdom; and to depart from evil is understanding.

• Psalms (read whole book, especially, 37:4) - Delight thyself also in the Lord; and he shall give thee the desires of thine heart.

• Proverbs 3:5-6 - Trust in the Lord with all thine heart; and lean not unto thine own understanding.   In all thy ways acknowledge him, and he shall direct thy paths. Counsel is mine, and sound wisdom, I am understanding; I have strength.

• Isaiah 49:16 - Behold, I have given thee upon the palms of my hands; the walls are continually before me. But he was wounded for our transgressions, he was bruised for our iniquities; the chastisement of our peace was upon him; and with this stripes we are healed. For my thoughts are not your thoughts, neither are your ways my ways, saith the Lord. For as the heavens are higher than the earth, so are my ways higher than your ways, and my thoughts than your thoughts.

• Ezekiel 16:6 (to stop severe bleeding, it still works now days) - And when I passed by thee, and saw thee polluted in thine own blood, I said unto thee when thou wast in thy blood, Live; yea, I said unto thee when thou wast in thy blood, Live.

• Matthew 3:11 - I indeed baptize you with water unto repentance; but he that cometh after me is mightier than I, whose shoes I am not worthy to bear; he shall baptize you with the Holy Ghost, and with fire.

Matthew 4:4-It is correctly written man shall not live by bread alone, but by every word that proceedeth out of the mouth of God.

Matthew 5:3-11

* Blessed are the poor in spirit; for theirs is the kingdom of heaven.

* Blessed are they that mourn; for they shall be comforted.

* Blessed are the meek; for they shall inherit the earth.

* Blessed are they which do hunger and thirst after righteousness; for they shall be filled.

* Blessed are the merciful; for they shall obtain mercy.

* Blessed are the pure in heart; for they shall see God.

* Blessed are the peacemakers; for they shall be called the children of God.

* Blessed are they which are persecuted for righteousness sake; for theirs is the kingdom of heaven.

* Blessed are ye, when men shall revile you and persecute you, and shall say all manner of evil against you falsely, my sake.

Matthew 5:38-48 - Ye have heard that it hath been said, an eye for an eye, and a tooth for a tooth: but I say unto you, that ye resist not evil: but whosoever shall smite thee on thy right cheek, turn to him the other also, and if any man will sue thee at the law, and take away thy coat, let hime have they cloak also. And whosoever shall compel thee to go a mile, go with him twain. Give to him that asketh thee and from him that would borrow of thee turn not thou away. Ye have heard that it hath been said, thou shalt love thy neighbor, and hate thine enemy. But I say unto you, Love your enemies, bless them that curse you, do good to them that hate you, and pray for them which despitefully use you, and persecute you; that ye may be the children of your Father which is in heaven: for he maketh his sun to rise on the evil and on the good, and sendeth rain on the just and on the unjust. For if ye love them which love you, what reward have ye? Do not even the publicans the same? And if ye salute your brethren only, what do ye more than others? Do not even the publicans so? Be ye therefore perfect, even as your Father which is in heaven is perfect.

Matthew 6:15 - But if ye forgive not men their trespasses, neither will your Father forgive your trespasses.

Matthew 7:12 - Therefore, all things whatsoever ye would that men should do to you, do ye even so to them: for this is the law and the prophets.

Matthew 10:26-42 - Fear them not therefore: for there is nothing covered, that shall not be revealed; and hid, that shall not be known. What I tell you in darkness, that speak ye in light: and what ye hear in the ear, that reach ye upon the housetops. And fear not them which kill the body, but are not able to kill the soul; but rather fear him which is able to destroy both soul and body in hell. Are not two sparrows sold for a farthing? And one of them shall not fall on the ground without your Father. But the very hairs of your head are all numbered. Fear ye not therefore, ye are of more value than many sparrows. Whosoever therefore shall confess me before men, him will I confess also before my Father which is in heaven. But whosoever shall deny me before men, him will I also deny before my Father which is in heaven. Think not that I am come to send peace on earth: I came not to send peace, but a sword. For I am come to set a man at variance against her mother, and the daughter-in-law against her mother-in-law and a mans foes shall be they of his own household. He that loveth father or mother more than me is not worthy of me: and he that loveth son or daughter more than me is not worthy of me. And he that taketh not his cross, and followeth after me, is not worthy of me. He that findeth his life shall lose it; and he that loseth his life for my sake shall find it. He that receiveth you receiveth me, and he that receiveth me receiveth him that sent me. He that receiveth a prophet in the mane of a prophet shall receive a prophets reward; and he that receiveth a righteous man in the name of a righteous man shall receive a righteous man's reward. And whosoever shall give to drink unto one of these little ones a cup of cold water only in the mane of a disciple, verily I say unto you, he shall in no way lose his reward. Matthew 11:5-6 - The blind receive their sight, and the lame walk, the lepers are cleansed, and the deaf hear, the dead are raised up, and the poor have the gospel preached to them.

And blessed is he, whosoever shall not be offended in me.

Matthew 12:22-31 - Then was brought unto him one possessed with a devil, blind and dumb: and he healed him, insomuch that the blind and dumb both spoke and saw. And all the people were amazed, and said, Is not this the son of David? But when the Pharisees heard it, they said, This fellow doth not cast out devils, but by Beelze-bub the prince of the devils. And Jesus knew their thoughts, and said unto them Every kingdom divided against itself is brought to desolation; and every city or house divided against itself shall not stand: and if Satan cast out Satan, he is divided against himself; how shall then his kingdom stand? And if I by Beelze-bub case out devils, by whom do your children cast them out? Therefore they shall be your judges. But if I cast out devils by the Spirit of God, then the kingdom of God is come unto you. Or else how can one enter into a strong man's house, and spoil his goods except he first bind the strong man? And then he will spoil his house. He that is not with me is against me; and he that gathereth not with me scattereth abroad.

Wherefore I say unto you, all manners of sins and blasphemy against the Holy Ghost shall not be forgiven unto men.

Matthew 16:3-4 - And verily I say unto you, except, ye be converted, and become as little children, ye shall not enter the kingdom of heaven. Whosoever therefore shall humble himself as this little child, the same is greatest in the kingdom of heaven.

Matthew 19:23-26 - Then said Jesus unto his disciples, Verily I say unto you, that a rich man shall hardly enter into the kingdom of heaven. And again I say unto you, It is easier for a camel to go through the eye of a needle, than for a rich man to enter into the kingdom of God. When his disciples heard it, they were exceedingly amazed, saying: who then can be saved? But Jesus beheld them, and said unto them, "With men this is impossible; but with God all things are possible.

• Mark 16:15-20 - And he said unto them, Go ye into all the world, and preach the gospel to every creature. He that believeth and is baptized shall be saved: but he that believeth not shall be damned. And these signs shall follow them that believe; In my name shall they cast out devils; they shall speak with new tongues; They shall take up serpents; and if they drink any deadly thing, it shall not hurt them; they shall lay hands on the sick, and they shall recover. So then after the Lord had spoken unto them, he was received up into heaven, and sat on the right hand of God. And they went forth, and preached everywhere, the Lord working with them and confirming the word with signs following. Amen.

• Luke 10:19 - Behold, I give unto you power to tread on serpents and scorpions, and over all power of the enemy; and nothing shall by any means hurt you. 23:34 - Then said Jesus, Father forgive them; for they know not what they do.

• John 3:5-7 - Jesus said; Verily, verily, I say unto thee, except a man be born of Water and of the Spirit, he cannot enter into the kingdom of God. That which is born of the flesh is flesh; and that which is born of the Spirit is spirit. Marvel not that I said unto thee, ye must be born again.

• John 13:13-14-If I then, your Lord and Master, have washed your feet; ye also ought to wash one another's feet. For I have given you an example, that ye should do as I have done to you.

• John 14:3 - I go and prepare a place for you, I will come again, and receive you unto myself; that where I am, there ye may be also.

• John 14:13 - And whatsoever ye shall ask in my name, that will I do, that the Father may be glorified in the Son.

• Acts 1: 8 - But ye shall receive power, after that the Holy Ghost is come upon you; and ye shall be witnesses unto me both in Jerusalem and in all Judea and in Samaria, and unto the uttermost part of the earth.

• Acts 4:12 - Neither is there salvation in any other: for there is none other name under heaven given among men, whereby we must be saved.

• Acts 11:16 - Then remembered I the word of the Lord, how that he said John indeed baptized with water; but ye shall be baptized with the Holy Ghost.

• Romans 1:17 - For therein is the righteousness of God revealed from faith to faith: as it is written, the just shall live by faith.

• Romans 8:17 - and if Children then heirs; heirs of God and joint-heirs with Christ, if so be that we suffer with him, that we are also glorified together.

• Romans 14:17 - For the kingdom of God is not meat and drink; but righteousness and peace, and joy in the Holy Ghost.

• Hebrews 4:12 - For the word of God is quick and powerful, sharper than any two-edged sword, piercing even to the dividing asunder of soul and spirit and of the joints and marrow, and is a discerner of the thoughts and intents of the heart.

• James 1:17 - Every good gift and every perfect gift is from above, and cometh down from the Father of lights, and whom is no variableness, neither shadow of turning.

• Jeremiah 32:27 – Behold, I am the Lord, the God of all flesh: Is there anything to hard for me?

• Psalms 46:10 – Be still and know I am God; I will be exalted among the heathen, I will be exalted in the earth.

• John 3:16 – Behold I stand at the door and knock (Open the door people for your own salvation)…..

*Note: Concerning all Holly Bible Scriptures, ***you must believe***.

Chapter 7
Deep Sincere Prayers;
My Animals a Sign?

You know how animals were used in the Old Testament as a sacrifice? No, I did not use my personal animals as a sacrificed and never will. There is no need to now. Jesus is our sacrifice, Our Lord has in the Bible "Not to worry about what too eat of how God feeds the birds and are not we more worthy than the birds?" Mathew 6:25-26. One time I had a hamster named Charlie. One day God spoke to me in the inner voice telling me to check on Charlie. When I went to check on Charlie, the Lord said: "Turn him over on his back". I must admit, I kind of wondered why our Lord Jesus told me that, but I did as Jesus said. Then I suddenly knew why Jesus told me. Charlie had a knot on his belly. I immediately took Charlie to the veterinarian. All the doctor had to do was look at Charlie. He immediately told me that Charlie had cancer. The doctor went on to say of that's why rats are used in medical research so much, since they get cancer a lot. I had the doctor put Charlie to sleep. I did not want him to suffer a agonizing death.

Then one time I had a dog name Sparky. One particular day I walked into my bedroom and found Sparky on my bed. Sparky was on his back and with all four paws sticking straight up. Sparky was hard as dried cement (like I already mentioned of how hard I would turn). He reminded me of an animal that had been dead on the side of the road for several days. I was walking out of my bedroom to tell my husband that Sparky was dead, when suddenly I thought I heard Sparky walking behind me in the hallway. I turned around and looked, sure enough Sparky was alive and well. I immediately called up the veterinarian and explained to the receptionist of what happened. I was shocked by what she told me. The receptionist said: "Sparky had a seizure." I said: "a seizure?" She went on to say: "Yes, dogs can have seizures like humans." I told her I was bringing Sparky in. When I arrived I had Sparky put to sleep. I did not want Charlie and Sparky to suffer.

Then when I had a certain brain test done, (before my surgery) it was called the Wada test. With this test each side of my brain was put to sleep, one side at a time. The same day I was scheduled for the Wada test, I woke up early in the morning in my home. I uncovered my cockatiels' cage (their names are Adam and Eve) and found Adam dead on his back. I found it mighty strange that I was scheduled to have my Wada test and Adam "went to sleep' in his own way. I would never hurt my animals or anyone. Before my surgery, I could not help to think over and over of what happened.

Then one particular scripture kept coming to my mind. The one that says that you are not to worry about what to eat. I just could not stop thinking about it. So, when I was in deep sincere prayer (before my surgery) for God's healing power, I kept telling Jesus of how he told me about Charlie. I also reminded

Jesus of Sparky and Adam. I especially told Jesus that was why I had put Charlie and Sparky to sleep. I did not want them to suffer. In my prayers I used the scripture Matthew 6: 25-26 a lot. I told the Lord Jesus: "Even though I loved my animals dearly Lord, are not I more worthy than them?" Surely, Lord Jesus, if me being sinful, and having mercy on my animals, would you not have more mercy on me (Especially after 46 years of suffering from having seizures)?

I find it hard to believe Adam just died. I believe with all my heart Jesus knew that I would use my animals in my prayers concerning my healing and that's why he allowed Charlie to get cancer, Sparky to have seizures, and Adam die naturally (How? I'll never know).

I know I miss and still love my animals dearly. Don't go around sacrificing your animals. Jesus became mankinds' sacrifice when he was nailed upon the cross. The Lord never even told me to put Charlie and Sparky to sleep. That was my own personal choice.

Thank you sweet Jesus, for your Love and Understanding!

Chapter 8
Time for Surgery

Readers of this book: This chapter will be short because I did not have much experience with it time-wise. Anyway, after 48 years of tormenting grand-mal seizures I had surgery that would either stop them all together or at least, hopefully, stop me from having so many.

Before I was operated on, the surgeons' assistant told me about a new 'product' they would like to use on me during the surgery for research purposes. It was a type of glue (like super glue) that was suppose to stop the stitches (they were going to use under the skin covering my brain) from 'leaking'. After 48 years of seizures and torment, I was willing to try anything. After all, I had reached a point in my life where I was desperate. Nothing else in my life had ever worked to stop me from having seizures, so I was willing to try just about anything. So after questioning her about what could/ would happen (side effects) I agreed to allow them to use the glue. It did not scare me in any way as I had put everything into the Lords' hands. I must admit that I did have some question as to whether the glue would make me high or what? But, after I had talked to the assistant I did agree to let them use me as a guinea pig and use the glue on my stitches. After all, I had put my trust in the Lord to guide and direct the surgeons' hands during the surgery. Then I got to thinking, what if the glue did not work and the stitches so happened to tear, then would my brain turn to rust? It may seem silly, but as a human that thought for some reason just started running through my head over and over again.

I certainly did not want my brain to turn to rust or dust (who would?). The doctor never said it would, but who knows what brought that thought about in me? I did sign a paper allowing the surgeon to use the glue and agree to follow-up appointments to allow them to check the area to see how it was holding up.

Anyway, after the surgery, the only 'high' I felt appeared to be from the anesthesia they used to put me to sleep. I had asked the surgeons' assistant if the glue would stay in my brain forever or what. (I do like to ask questions, especially after trying so many different 'remedies' to stop seizures over the 48 prior years). At that time, three months of my surgery had gone by, the assistant told me that the glue would be coming out through my urine. I thank Jesus daily that he had the Holy Spirit guide me into making the right decision. Of course, whatever your situation is, it will be up to you and your doctor(s).

As of April 13, 2004, five months since my surgery, I had not had any more seizures. Since that time, however, I have started having them again, but am not having them as often as I had in the past and Praise be to God, most have not been as severe as some I've had in the past. I do highly recommend a neurologist and neurosurgeon for this surgery and pray with all my heart the Jesus will guide any other epileptics who have considered having this type of surgery to strongly consider having it. Talk to your doctors, pray to the Lord and ask for his divine guidance.

I truly believe this information needs to be gotten out quickly. Therefore, I need to get this book published as fast as possible.

God bless you all richly. I can not ever stop telling or writing it enough.

In Jesus Name,

Joanne Curry

Chapter 9
After Surgery

After the surgery, the surgeon was slapping me real hard on my right hand saying: "Wake up Joanne, the surgery is over with". I could hear the surgeon and everyone talking, but I had some trouble waking up. "Wow, was that anesthesia strong". That's fine, I didn't really want to wake up during surgery.

In fact, I had previously asked the surgeon if it would be possible for me to go into a seizure during surgery. He said: "No way, because your brain is put to sleep". I eventually very slowly turned my head towards my right side. In 'fuzziness' when I came awake, I first saw what looked like a woman to me. I suddenly got so happy, so excited. You know like how a child is so happy to see their mommy, daddy, grandpa, grandma, or go to the zoo?

I suddenly (or should I say miraculously felt like a little excited child, I felt so humble!). The next thing I knew I asked: "Are you Jeeeeeesus?" (I spelled Jesus's name that way, because that was how I pronounced his name). I now believe without a doubt it was because I knew in my sub-conscious Jesus was there. At that time (in the surgery room) I honestly thought it was because I was so high, due to the anesthesia).

The lady answered me: (laughing in a respectful, loving laugh) "No, honey, I'm not Jesus". Then she again laughed respectfully and said: "No, honey, I'm DEFINETELY NOT JESUS!!!!!" I had to be monitored in the intensive care unit (ICU) for 24 hours after the surgery for them to keep a constant check on me for swelling or bleeding of my brain.

All turned out okay. I knew in my heart Jesus was with me all the way! I was then moved to my regular hospital room. A patient (after brain surgery) is usually in the hospital three to five days. The first time the surgeon who operated on me walked into my hospital room he looked at me: and immediately said to me: "You just finished having major surgery". I remember very clearly of how I gave him a look like: "Why are you telling me this, I know". (I'll explain a little later of why I looked at the surgeon that way).

Most of you readers will probably think I was so high I didn't know what was happening to me. It was only the second day of me being in the hospital. As you probably already know, I was hooked up to all sorts of monitors with wires and I had a catheter in me. A technician came in to check on me, especially my catheter. He mainly seemed to be most concerned about how I looked. Well, I guess I looked great to him. He did not say anything to me he just took out the catheter and left the hospital room.

About twenty to thirty minutes later a different male technician came into my hospital room. He immediately noticed my catheter had been removed. He said: "Oh I see they took out your catheter. How are you going to the bathroom, using your bedpan?" I took notice of how he had a half smirk and a sort of smiling look on his face. I looked at him like: "How do you think?" I then said: (smirking back at him) "No, I'm getting up and walking to the bath room on my own".

If only all of you readers could have seen the look on his face. He suddenly opened his eyes very wide and his mouth was hanging opened. By the look on his face, I knew he was going to tell the surgeon (especially since he very quickly left my hospital room). Then about twenty minutes later the surgeon walks back into my room not even questioning me as to how I was doing, how I was feeling or even telling me: 'Hello Joanne'. Oh, I guess I forgive him (I was only joking about his not showing any concern). He did nothing wrong or disrespectful. He is a neurosurgeon with lots of understanding love, mercy and humbleness! This is what I meant by him never even saying "hello" to me. He mentioned to me: "You know Joanne, there are a lot of people who come out of brain surgery that can not walk, talk or even get out of the bed. Here you are doing everything yourself!"

As I already mentioned, I was going to the bathroom, giving myself sponge baths (obviously I could not get into the shower because of all the wires, IV hook-ups, etc.). I was even feeding myself and walking up and down the hallway. I know without a doubt that the doctor knew it was a miracle. He did not expect me to be able to do all the things I was doing for myself.

He did not even expect me to realize I just had brain surgery. That's why he told me about just finishing having major surgery. My surgeon, last by not least, told me: "I want a cat scan of your brain". When the result from the cat scan came back, the surgeon returned. He was amazed and told me: "Your brain is healing so fast, there is absolutely no reason for you to stay here in this hospital any longer. You can go home." This was after being out of surgery for only 24 hours.

I immediately asked him: "When am I going home?" He told me: "Today, right after lunch!" Wouldn't you know it my church sister (Renee) had called me right after the surgeon walked out. She mentioned to me that she and our pastor's wife (Mother

McCloud) wanted to come out to visit me (may I add, it is about an hour drive just one way, just for them to visit). I happily told her: "Do not waste your time, I am going home!" Sister Renee was so amazed and happy for me.

(NOTE: Even though I believe without a doubt that the neurologist and neurosurgeon are extremely skilled and highly proficient professionals, I prefer not to mention their names. I have my reason for not naming them. All I will say as I mentioned earlier, I had my brain surgery in Tampa, Florida).

Chapter 10
My Prayer for You

Jesus, first I ask You for forgiveness so I can be more worthy and holy in thy sight. As you know Lord, I suffered with my grand mal convulsions 48 years. Remember Lord all the convulsions I had? Remember Lord the many, many, times I was having grand-mal's every 2-3 hours, for two, three, four, and at times five days straight?

As you know Jesus it was discovered by the neurosurgeon the "night-light" on the right side of my brain was so bright (that's what the surgeon explained to me and called it the 'night-light'). Due to the extra brightness of this 'night light' it was causing something like 'anger' to go through my brain. Lord, it is utterly amazing that I am even still alive. I am an actual walking miracle, Lord. Praise be to Thy most Holy Name.

Jesus, after all the grand mal seizures I had after 48 years, haven't I suffered enough for not only myself, but as others with seizures have also endured?   I know their physical and emotional pains Lord. I know their torments Lord. Please Jesus do not let my 48 years of torment be for nothing.

Lord Jesus, your word says: "Ask anything in my name and I will do it"-John 14:14.'). I ask in your name Jesus, that you will heal all epileptics. It doesn't matter how you do it Lord, absolutely divinely or through a neurosurgeon. All I ask Lord Jesus is that You heal them. Let the power of the Holy Spirit build up their faith to where they will be utterly amazed. I could not give up my faith. Lord, I had to keep believing. What would I have gained by giving up? Please, please, sweet and loving Lord Jesus, have mercy on them and on myself.

For the ones that have given up, allow the power of my faith that I had then (*and still do be on their behalf.*) My dear merciful, loving, sweet Jesus, please do not forget the 48 years I was tormented. Allow all the torments I went through to also be on their behalf. Have not I suffered enough for all epileptics or others with seizures?

All I can really do Lord Jesus is basically believe for them (again) on their behalf and ask you in your name, Jesus. I thank you with all my heart Lord. You know how much I appreciate all you have done for me. Bless all epileptics and all the medical personnel who work so hard to care for us all in need. Send more surgeons and understanding medical personnel to all epileptics in need of help.

I love you Lord Jesus. In your name Jesus, Amen.

Let the words of my mouth and the meditation of my heart be acceptable in thy sight, oh Lord, my strength and my redeemer. (Psalms 19:14) In your name, Jesus.

Surgery may not be for everyone. It is not always a guarantee to solve ones problems. Before considering any surgery, not just for seizures, one should pray extensively for

Jesus' guidance and discuss all concerns with your regular doctor and with the surgeon who will be performing the procedure.

As for myself, I am ever so thankful that the Lord guided me to go through with the surgery. It has not been a cure-all, but it has helped. I thank Jesus for all of his divine help in guiding the surgeons hands and in my continuing recovery.

Special Thanks To:

Pastor Ira J. McCloud and Mother Pirieta McCloud for being my pastor and spiritual parents.

Minister Kasseem Weston for helping me find some biblical scriptures.

Minister Ronnie Strickland for baptizing my daughter Jennifer Marie.

Minister Josh for assisting me in finding biblical scriptures.

Sister Stacey Wesley for being a special counselor for me (especially for understanding my deep hurt and anger).

Sister Janice Brantley for the times we enjoyed going out to eat after church services.

Sister Renee 0. Veasy for always making me feel good again, to laugh and for typing up my papers for this book.

Sister Barbara for always being a friend and calling to check on me.

A special thank you to EVERYONE at Refuge Church of Our Lord, for being my brothers & Sisters in Christ.

For more information call the Refuge Church of Our Lord — 642 Harris Street/P.O. Box 3831 Sebring, FL 33871-3071. (863) 382-1855.

Authorhouse for publishing this work.

Most of all the Lord Jesus Christ in whom all things are possible.

Special Forgiveness, Mercy, Love and Peace from our Lord Jesus Christ

Extra Special Thanks To:

Bruce, my husband for bearing with me, especially concerning the stress he goes through and has went through with me having seizures. Also, if it had not been for him and his love, I would never have been able to make it so far.

My mother, Isabel. All the things she went through on earth having to deal with my illness over these many years.

But most of all; THE LORD JESUS CHRIST, for guiding me in writing this book. Thank you! In Jesus name.

About the Author

Joanne P. Curry is fifty (50) years old, and has lived in Florida for most of her life. She has been an epileptic for forty-eight (48) years.